LOW POTASSIUM

FOOD LIST

The Complete Ingredient list and

Food to Avoid For Low

Potassium Diet

Harley W. Norman

Table of Contents

Introduction

"Are You Tired of the Constant Worry Over Your Potassium Levels?"

Every day, millions of people struggle with the balancing act of maintaining healthy potassium levels. Whether you're dealing with kidney issues, heart problems, or just striving for a healthier lifestyle, the constant monitoring of what you eat can feel overwhelming. Isn't it time you found a simpler way to live well without the worry?

Discover the Freedom of a Low Potassium Lifestyle

Our comprehensive guide, **"Low Potassium Food List"**, is meticulously crafted to offer you peace of mind and freedom in your dietary choices. Here's what you'll gain from our book:

- **Freedom from Confusion**: Clearly outlined lists of what to eat and what to avoid, freeing you from the hassle of guesswork.

- **Improved Health and Wellbeing**: Learn how managing your potassium intake can alleviate symptoms related to high potassium levels, enhancing your overall health.

- **Diverse and Delicious Recipes**: Delight in a variety of recipes that cater to low potassium needs without sacrificing flavor.

- **Practical Tips for Everyday Life**: From grocery shopping to dining out, our book covers all bases, making your new dietary habits easy and sustainable.

Addressing Your Concerns

"But isn't a low potassium diet incredibly restrictive?" While it's true that managing your diet can sometimes feel limiting, our book is designed to expand your culinary horizons. We provide you with numerous food alternatives and innovative recipes that keep your meals exciting and varied.

"I worry I won't be able to stick to a low potassium diet." Change can be daunting, but our guide is equipped with practical meal plans, tips for eating out, and support resources that make sticking to your new diet manageable and stress-free.

By choosing **"Low Potassium Food List"**, you're not just buying a book; you're gaining a lifelong companion in your journey toward better health. Embrace the opportunity to transform your dietary habits and enhance your life quality with confidence. Start your journey today, worry-free!

Understanding Potassium

Potassium is an essential mineral that plays a crucial role in the functioning of the human body, affecting everything from nerve transmission to muscle contraction, including the vital function of the heart. It helps regulate fluid balance, aids in the transmission of nerve signals, and helps muscles contract properly. The importance of potassium extends to its role in maintaining a healthy blood pressure level, and it also supports proper heart rhythms.

Despite its benefits, the management of potassium intake is critical, especially for individuals with certain health conditions. For those with compromised kidney function, maintaining a low potassium diet becomes essential because their kidneys may not be able to remove excess potassium effectively. High potassium levels in the blood, a condition known as hyperkalemia, can lead to dangerous health issues, including cardiac arrhythmia or even a heart attack.

In the context of a low potassium food list, it's important to understand that the average adult needs about 2,600 to 3,400 milligrams of potassium per day. Foods rich in potassium include bananas, oranges, potatoes, and spinach, which may need to be limited or avoided on a low potassium diet. Instead, options like apples, berries, cabbage, and cauliflower are recommended as they are naturally lower in potassium.

For those managing their potassium intake, the challenge often lies in balancing enough intake to maintain health while avoiding excess that can exacerbate existing conditions. This requires not only knowledge of which foods are high and low in potassium but also an understanding of how to read food labels and recognize the potassium content in ingredients that are less obvious.

The ability to manage and adjust dietary potassium is a skill that can significantly impact the health and wellbeing of individuals needing to follow a low potassium diet. This management is facilitated by resources like the "Low Potassium Food List," which provide vital information to navigate this dietary requirement efficiently. Such resources empower individuals to make informed choices about their diets, leading to improved health outcomes and a better quality of life while living with dietary restrictions related to potassium.

Importance of Managing Potassium Intake

Potassium is a vital mineral that plays several crucial roles in the body, including regulating fluid balance, maintaining proper nerve functions, and facilitating muscle contractions, including those in the heart. Despite its importance, both excessive and insufficient potassium levels can lead to serious health complications, making the management of potassium intake essential, especially for individuals with certain medical conditions.

For those with kidney disease, the kidneys may not be able to remove excess potassium efficiently. This can lead to hyperkalemia, a condition characterized by dangerously high levels of potassium in the blood, which can cause muscle weakness, paralysis, and life-threatening heart irregularities. Conversely, insufficient potassium, or hypokalemia, can lead to fatigue, muscle cramps, and cardiovascular problems. Managing potassium intake is crucial in preventing these extreme fluctuations that can severely impact overall health.

A low potassium food list serves as a vital tool for individuals who need to monitor and adjust their potassium intake closely. By clearly outlining which foods are low in potassium, the list helps in making informed dietary choices to maintain balanced potassium levels. For instance, instead of high potassium foods like bananas, oranges, and potatoes, the list suggests alternatives like apples, berries, and cauliflower, which contribute to nutritional needs without the risk of increasing potassium to a dangerous level.

Moreover, understanding which foods to limit or avoid is just as important as knowing safe alternatives. This detailed guidance helps individuals avoid the common pitfalls of dietary management, such as unknowingly consuming foods rich in potassium that are often hidden in processed goods and restaurant meals.

In managing potassium intake, the goal is not only to avoid immediate health risks but also to maintain long-term health and prevent the complications associated with imbalanced electrolyte levels. Regular consultation of a low potassium food list simplifies this task, empowering individuals to make choices that support their health without constant worry or complication. This proactive approach to diet can significantly enhance the quality of life for those dealing with potassium management issues, providing them with a greater sense of control over their health and wellbeing.

Overview of Low Potassium Diet

A low potassium diet is crucial for individuals who need to manage their potassium intake due to certain health conditions, such as kidney disease or heart ailments. This type of diet helps in maintaining potassium levels within a safe range, thereby preventing potential health complications. In essence, the diet involves limiting the consumption of foods that are high in potassium, which is a mineral essential for proper functioning of the nerves and muscles, including the heart.

Potassium is naturally present in many fruits, vegetables, dairy products, and meats. While a typical diet might encourage high intakes of fruits and vegetables like bananas, oranges, and potatoes, a low potassium diet requires avoiding these and opting for alternatives that have lower potassium content. For instance, instead of bananas, a person might eat apples; instead of potatoes, white rice or cauliflower might be preferable.

The goal of this diet is not just about avoiding high potassium foods but also about balancing intake to avoid both excessive and too little potassium, as both extremes can have serious health implications. For instance, high potassium levels can lead to hyperkalemia, a condition that can cause nausea, weakness, and even life-threatening heart arrhythmias. On the other hand, insufficient potassium can lead to hypokalemia, presenting risks such as fatigue, muscle cramps, and cardiovascular problems.

Adherence to a low potassium diet also extends to how food is prepared. For example, certain cooking methods, such as leaching and boiling vegetables before eating them, can help reduce their potassium content. The dietary plan should be well-rounded and nutritionally balanced to ensure that all other nutritional needs are met, considering that restricting potassium might inadvertently lower the intake of other important nutrients.

Meal planning on a low potassium diet involves careful consideration and knowledge of the potassium content in various foods. This is where a comprehensive guide like "Low Potassium Food List" comes into play. It provides detailed lists of suitable foods and those to avoid. It also offers meal suggestions and recipes that fit into a low potassium diet, making it easier for individuals to adhere to their dietary restrictions without sacrificing taste or nutritional value.

Furthermore, this diet is not static and the amount of potassium permitted can vary depending on the individual's health status, kidney function, and treatment goals. Regular consultation with healthcare providers is essential to tailor the diet appropriately and monitor potassium levels to ensure they remain within the target range.

Overall, a low potassium diet, when followed correctly and consistently, helps in managing and preventing the complications associated with abnormal potassium levels, ultimately supporting better long-term health outcomes.

Understanding Your Daily Potassium Needs

Recommended Daily Allowance for Potassium

The recommended daily allowance (RDA) for potassium varies depending on age, gender, and life stage. Generally, adults should aim for about 2,600 to 3,400 milligrams per day. Specifically, adult women need approximately 2,600 milligrams, while adult men should consume about 3,400 milligrams of potassium daily. These values can serve as a guide for healthy individuals without kidney problems or conditions that affect potassium metabolism.

For those following a low potassium diet due to health conditions such as chronic kidney disease (CKD), the daily intake may need to be significantly lower. Healthcare professionals often recommend these individuals limit their potassium to between 800 and 2,000 milligrams per day, depending on the severity of their condition and their specific health needs. It is crucial for these patients to work closely with a dietitian or a healthcare provider to determine an appropriate intake level that safely manages their condition without leading to other health issues.

Children and teenagers have different requirements based on their rapid growth and development stages. Children between the ages of 1 and 3 should consume about 2,000 milligrams per day, those between 4 and 8 years old require about 2,300 milligrams, and from ages 9 to 13, the recommendation increases to about 2,500 milligrams. Teenagers between the ages of 14 and 18 should aim for about 2,600 milligrams for females and 3,000 milligrams for males.

Pregnant and lactating women have increased needs for potassium to support fetal growth and milk production. Pregnant women are advised to consume about 2,900 milligrams per day, while lactating women should aim for approximately 2,800 milligrams daily.

Understanding these recommendations is crucial for anyone managing their potassium intake, especially when adhering to a low potassium diet. The "Low Potassium Food List" provides a vital resource, detailing food options that are appropriate for maintaining a lower potassium intake. This resource can be incredibly helpful for meal planning and ensuring that daily potassium intake remains within the recommended limits tailored to individual health requirements. This tailored approach helps prevent the complications associated with both high and low potassium levels, such as muscle weakness, heart irregularities, and potentially life-threatening conditions. Regular monitoring of potassium levels through blood tests is also essential to ensure that dietary adjustments are effective and safe.

Factors Affecting Potassium Needs

Several factors influence individual potassium needs, making it important to understand these variables when managing potassium intake, especially for those who require a low potassium diet. One of the primary factors is the overall health of the kidneys. The kidneys play a crucial role in regulating potassium levels by filtering and controlling the amount of potassium that is excreted in the urine. People with chronic kidney disease or other renal impairments may not be able to process potassium efficiently, which can lead to an accumulation in the blood, necessitating a lower potassium intake.

Age is another significant factor. Older adults often have decreased kidney function and may take medications that affect potassium levels, such as certain diuretics or blood pressure drugs. These medications can increase the risk of hyperkalemia (high potassium levels), thereby adjusting the amount of potassium that should be consumed.

The overall health condition of an individual also plays a role. Conditions such as diabetes and heart disease can influence how the body handles potassium. For instance, insulin and certain heart medications can affect potassium metabolism, influencing dietary needs. People with these conditions often need to monitor their potassium intake more closely to avoid complications.

Activity level and physical health are additional determinants of potassium needs. Athletes or those who engage in vigorous physical activity lose electrolytes, including potassium, through sweat. This can increase their dietary potassium requirements. However, if someone is less active, particularly if they have underlying health issues that affect potassium regulation, they may need to limit their intake.

Dietary habits also affect potassium levels. Consuming large amounts of processed foods, which are often low in potassium, might seem beneficial for those needing to restrict their intake. However, these foods can also be high in sodium, which can affect potassium levels indirectly by influencing kidney function and fluid retention.

Hormonal changes and conditions can alter potassium needs as well. For example, conditions like Addison's disease (a disorder of the adrenal glands) can lead to increased potassium retention, necessitating adjustments in dietary intake.

Genetic factors may also play a role. Some genetic conditions can affect the body's ability to process potassium properly, which might require tailored dietary guidelines to manage potassium levels effectively.

Finally, environmental factors such as climate and weather can also influence potassium needs. In hot climates, for example, individuals may lose more potassium through sweat and may need to adjust their intake accordingly if they do not have conditions that require potassium restriction.

Understanding these factors is crucial for anyone managing their potassium levels through diet. It helps in customizing dietary choices to meet personal health needs effectively, ensuring that the body maintains a healthy potassium balance. This approach underscores the importance of a resource like "Low Potassium Food List," which provides guidance tailored to varying needs and circumstances, helping individuals make informed dietary choices.

Symptoms of High Potassium Levels

High potassium levels in the blood, known medically as hyperkalemia, can be a silent condition, often presenting minimal or no symptoms until the levels are significantly elevated. When symptoms do occur, they are typically related to the effects of potassium on the electrical activity of the heart and the neuromuscular functions of the body.

The initial symptoms of hyperkalemia can be quite subtle and may include a general feeling of fatigue or weakness. As potassium levels continue to rise, the symptoms become more pronounced and can affect various bodily functions. One of the most serious impacts of high potassium levels is on the heart. Individuals may experience changes in their heart rhythm, which can feel like skipped heartbeats, palpitations, or an irregular pulse. In severe cases, dangerously high potassium can lead to sudden and serious changes in heart rhythm that can be life-threatening.

Muscle symptoms are also common and can range from mild weakness to severe paralysis. Initially, individuals might notice a tingling sensation or numbness in their limbs, or a fluttering feeling in the muscles. This can progress to muscle stiffness or cramping, and eventually to more pronounced muscle weakness. This weakness typically starts in the legs and can spread to other parts of the body, making movements difficult.

Neurological symptoms can include a feeling of numbness or tingling, particularly around the lips and fingers. Some people report a sense of mental fog, difficulty thinking clearly, or feeling lightheaded or dizzy. These symptoms arise because high potassium levels affect the way nerves transmit signals.

In extreme cases, if the potassium levels become critically high, it can lead to respiratory depression, where the muscles involved in breathing become too weak to function properly, posing a risk of respiratory failure.

Given these potential risks, it is vital for individuals at risk of hyperkalemia, such as those with kidney disease or those taking certain medications that affect kidney function, to manage their potassium intake effectively. This management is where resources like the "Low Potassium Food List" are invaluable. By providing detailed information on foods that are lower in potassium, this resource helps individuals make informed dietary choices to prevent the escalation of potassium levels in their bloodstream. Regular monitoring of potassium levels through blood tests is also crucial to ensure that they remain within a safe range, allowing timely dietary adjustments and medical interventions if necessary.

Maintaining potassium levels within the recommended range through careful dietary management not only helps mitigate the symptoms associated with hyperkalemia but also contributes to overall cardiovascular health and neuromuscular function.

Foods Low in Potassium

Fruits to Eat

For individuals following a low potassium diet, choosing the right fruits is essential as they can play a significant role in managing potassium levels while still providing necessary nutrients.

Fruit	Serving Size	Potassium Content	Calories	Other Nutrients	Preparation Tips
Apple	1 medium	195 mg	95 kcal	4g fiber, vitamin C	Eat raw, sliced, or add to salads
Pear	1 medium	206 mg	102 kcal	6g fiber, vitamin C	Fresh or canned in juice, not syrup
Blueberries	1 cup	114 mg	84 kcal	4g fiber, vitamin K, vitamin C	Fresh or frozen without added sugar

Fruit	Serving Size	Potassium Content	Calories	Other Nutrients	Preparation Tips
Strawberry	1 cup halves	254 mg	49 kcal	3g fiber, more vitamin C than oranges	Fresh or frozen, great for smoothies or salads
Peach	1 medium	285 mg	59 kcal	2g fiber, vitamin A, vitamin C	Fresh or canned in water
Blackberries	1 cup	233 mg	62 kcal	8g fiber, vitamin C, vitamin K	Fresh or frozen, ideal for desserts
Pineapple	1 cup chunks	180 mg	82 kcal	2g fiber, vitamin C, manganese	Fresh or grilled for a tropical dessert
Plum	1 medium	104 mg	30 kcal	1g fiber, vitamin C	Fresh or stewed
Clementine	1 medium	131 mg	35 kcal	Vitamin C, calcium	Fresh, peeled, or added to fruit salads

Fruit	Serving Size	Potassium Content	Calories	Other Nutrients	Preparation Tips
Raspberries	1 cup	186 mg	64 kcal	8g fiber, vitamin C, manganese	Fresh or frozen, perfect for topping yogurt
Cranberries	1 cup	85 mg	46 kcal	4g fiber, vitamin C, manganese	Fresh, dried without sugar, or as a juice blend
Cherries	1 cup	306 mg	97 kcal	3g fiber, vitamin C	Fresh, pitted for snacks or desserts
Grapes	1 cup	288 mg	62 kcal	1g fiber, vitamin C, vitamin K	Fresh, frozen as a cool snack
Watermelon	1 cup diced	170 mg	46 kcal	Vitamin A, vitamin C, hydration	Fresh, sliced, or diced for a hydrating treat
Lemon	1 medium	80 mg	17 kcal	Vitamin C, vitamin B6	Fresh, squeezed

Fruit	Serving Size	Potassium Content	Calories	Other Nutrients	Preparation Tips
					juice, zest for flavoring
Lime	1 medium	68 mg	20 kcal	Vitamin C, flavonoids	Fresh, squeezed juice, zest for cocktails
Tangerine	1 medium	132 mg	47 kcal	Vitamin C, vitamin A	Fresh, segments for salads or snacks
Apricot	1 medium	90 mg	17 kcal	Vitamin A, vitamin C	Fresh, dried without added sugars
Honeydew Melon	1 cup diced	388 mg	61 kcal	Vitamin C, copper	Fresh, cubed or balled for a sweet snack
Papaya	1 cup cubes	286 mg	55 kcal	3g fiber, vitamin C, vitamin A	Fresh, cubed or used in smoothies

This table provides a clear guide for incorporating low potassium fruits into a daily diet. Always consider the serving size and preparation method to ensure potassium levels are kept in check. These fruits offer a variety of flavors and nutritional benefits, making it easy to enjoy a diverse and satisfying low potassium diet.

Vegetables to Eat

Vegetable	Ingredient Details	Nutritional Information (per serving)	Serving Size	Cooking Time
Alfalfa sprouts	Fresh, raw	10 calories, 0.1g potassium	1 cup	None (raw)
Asparagus	Fresh, tips only	20 calories, 90mg potassium	6 spears	4-7 minutes
Bell peppers	Fresh, red or green	25 calories, 88mg potassium	1 cup sliced	5-10 minutes
Cabbage	Fresh, green or red	22 calories, 119mg potassium	1 cup shredded	5-10 minutes
Cauliflower	Fresh	25 calories, 88mg potassium	1 cup florets	5-10 minutes
Cucumber	Fresh, peeled	8 calories, 76mg potassium	½ cup sliced	None (raw)
Eggplant	Fresh	20 calories, 123mg potassium	1 cup cubed	15-20 minutes
Green beans	Fresh, trimmed	31 calories, 102mg potassium	1 cup	5-10 minutes
Iceberg	Fresh	10 calories, 102mg	1 cup	None

Vegetable	Ingredient Details	Nutritional Information (per serving)	Serving Size	Cooking Time
lettuce		potassium	shredded	(raw)
Mushrooms	Fresh, white	15 calories, 108mg potassium	1 cup sliced	5-10 minutes
Onions	Fresh, yellow	40 calories, 116mg potassium	½ cup chopped	10-15 minutes
Parsnips	Fresh	100 calories, 375mg potassium	1 cup sliced	10-15 minutes
Peas	Fresh, green	62 calories, 88mg potassium	½ cup	5-8 minutes
Radishes	Fresh	9 calories, 135mg potassium	10 radishes	None (raw)
Rhubarb	Fresh, without leaves	26 calories, 288mg potassium	1 cup diced	10-15 minutes
Turnips	Fresh, roots	34 calories, 124mg potassium	1 cup cubed	20-30 minutes
Water chestnuts	Fresh, peeled	40 calories, 350mg potassium	½ cup sliced	None (raw)
Zucchini	Fresh	20 calories, 180mg potassium	1 cup	5-10

Vegetable	Ingredient Details	Nutritional Information (per serving)	Serving Size	Cooking Time
		potassium	sliced	minutes
Endive	Fresh	8 calories, 157mg potassium	1 cup chopped	None (raw)
Collard greens	Fresh	30 calories, 83mg potassium	1 cup chopped	10-15 minutes

Each vegetable listed can be prepared in a variety of ways, such as raw, steamed, or sautéed, depending on your preference. The nutritional information and cooking times provided aim to help those managing their potassium intake to easily incorporate these vegetables into their meals. It's always a good idea to consult with a healthcare provider or a dietitian when making significant changes to your diet, especially for managing health conditions.

Grains and Bread Products

Ingredient	Preparation Instructions	Nutritional Information (per serving)	Serving Size	Cooking Time
White Rice	Boil in water until tender and fluffy.	68 mg potassium, 121 calories	1/2 cup cooked	18-20 minutes
White Bread	Toast or use fresh for sandwiches.	35 mg potassium, 66 calories	1 slice	N/A
Corn Flakes	Serve with low-potassium milk alternative like rice milk.	20 mg potassium, 100 calories	1 cup	N/A
Couscous	Boil in water or broth until water is absorbed and grains are fluffy.	58 mg potassium, 176 calories	1/2 cup cooked	5-10 minutes
Macaroni	Boil until al dente, rinse under cold water to stop cooking.	44 mg potassium, 221 calories	1/2 cup cooked	8-10 minutes

Ingredient	Preparation Instructions	Nutritional Information (per serving)	Serving Size	Cooking Time
Rice Noodles	Soak in hot water until soft, then drain.	14 mg potassium, 96 calories	1/2 cup cooked	8-10 minutes
Spaghetti (white)	Boil until al dente, rinse under cold water to stop cooking.	42 mg potassium, 220 calories	1/2 cup cooked	10-12 minutes
White Bagel	Toast and serve with low-potassium spreads.	70 mg potassium, 157 calories	1 small bagel	N/A
Pita Bread (white)	Toast lightly and serve.	49 mg potassium, 165 calories	1 small pita	N/A
Cornbread	Bake according to recipe, use low-potassium ingredients.	26 mg potassium, 198 calories	1 small piece	20-25 minutes
Plain Crackers	Serve with low-potassium cheese	21 mg potassium, 80	5 crackers	N/A

Ingredient	Preparation Instructions	Nutritional Information (per serving)	Serving Size	Cooking Time
	or spreads.	calories		
Sourdough Bread	Toast or serve fresh with meals.	30 mg potassium, 79 calories	1 slice	N/A
Pancakes (made from scratch using low-potassium recipe)	Cook on a hot griddle until golden brown.	50 mg potassium, 86 calories	1 pancake	10 minutes
English Muffins (white)	Toast and serve with suitable toppings.	37 mg potassium, 134 calories	1 muffin	N/A
Graham Crackers	Serve as a snack or use in recipes.	24 mg potassium, 59 calories	2 crackers	N/A
Pretzels (unsalted)	Serve as a snack.	40 mg potassium, 108 calories	1 oz	N/A

Ingredient	Preparation Instructions	Nutritional Information (per serving)	Serving Size	Cooking Time
Tortillas (white)	Heat and use for wraps or soft tacos.	32 mg potassium, 94 calories	1 medium	1-2 minutes
Farina (Cream of Wheat)	Cook in water or low-potassium milk alternative until thick.	35 mg potassium, 133 calories	3 tbsp dry	10 minutes
Rye Bread (light)	Toast or use for sandwiches.	70 mg potassium, 83 calories	1 slice	N/A
Oat Bran Muffins	Bake using low-potassium ingredients.	44 mg potassium, 128 calories	1 muffin	15-20 minutes

This table offers a variety of low-potassium grains and bread products that can be incorporated into a diet for those needing to manage their potassium levels. Each product listed provides alternatives that help maintain dietary variety and enjoyment while adhering to health guidelines.

Meats and Protein

When following a low potassium diet, choosing the right meats and proteins is crucial since some types of meat and protein sources can be high in potassium.

Ingredient	Cooking Instructions	Nutritional Information (per serving)	Serving Size	Cooking Time
Chicken breast, skinless	Grill or bake until the meat reaches an internal temperature of 165°F.	165 calories, 0g carbs, 31g protein, 3.6g fat, 256mg potassium	3 oz (85g)	20-25 minutes
Turkey breast, skinless	Roast in the oven at 325°F until the internal temperature reaches 165°F.	125 calories, 0g carbs, 26g protein, 1g fat, 210mg potassium	3 oz (85g)	30-40 minutes
Pork loin, lean	Roast at 375°F until the internal	190 calories, 0g carbs, 28g	3 oz (85g)	25 minutes

Ingredient	Cooking Instructions	Nutritional Information (per serving)	Serving Size	Cooking Time
	temperature reaches 145°F.	protein, 8g fat, 340mg potassium		
Veal, lean cut	Pan-fry or grill until well-cooked.	170 calories, 0g carbs, 25g protein, 7g fat, 310mg potassium	3 oz (85g)	6-8 minutes per side
Beef sirloin, trimmed	Grill or broil to desired doneness.	160 calories, 0g carbs, 25g protein, 7g fat, 280mg potassium	3 oz (85g)	10-12 minutes
Rabbit, cooked	Roast at 350°F until fully cooked.	147 calories, 0g carbs, 28g protein, 3g fat, 255mg potassium	3 oz (85g)	1 hour
Lamb loin, trimmed	Roast or grill until the internal	172 calories, 0g carbs, 24g	3 oz (85g)	15-20 minutes

Ingredient	Cooking Instructions	Nutritional Information (per serving)	Serving Size	Cooking Time
	temperature reaches 145°F for medium rare.	protein, 8g fat, 230mg potassium		
Duck, skin removed	Roast at 350°F until the internal temperature reaches 165°F.	140 calories, 0g carbs, 27g protein, 3g fat, 220mg potassium	3 oz (85g)	1.5 hours
Quail, cooked	Roast at 375°F until fully cooked.	123 calories, 0g carbs, 25g protein, 2g fat, 218mg potassium	1 quail	30 minutes
Venison, lean	Grill or broil until it reaches desired doneness.	134 calories, 0g carbs, 26g protein, 2g fat, 315mg potassium	3 oz (85g)	10 minutes
Cod, baked	Bake at 400°F	89 calories, 0g	3 oz	10-12

Ingredient	Cooking Instructions	Nutritional Information (per serving)	Serving Size	Cooking Time
	until fish flakes easily with a fork.	carbs, 20g protein, 1g fat, 244mg potassium	(85g)	minutes
Tilapia, baked	Bake at 375°F until opaque and moist.	110 calories, 0g carbs, 23g protein, 2g fat, 204mg potassium	3 oz (85g)	10-12 minutes
Flounder, baked	Bake at 350°F until fish is flaky.	99 calories, 0g carbs, 21g protein, 1g fat, 280mg potassium	3 oz (85g)	10-15 minutes
Trout, grilled	Grill over medium heat until cooked through.	128 calories, 0g carbs, 18g protein, 5g fat, 250mg potassium	3 oz (85g)	4-5 minutes per side
Haddock,	Bake at 350°F	95 calories, 0g	3 oz	10-15

Ingredient	Cooking Instructions	Nutritional Information (per serving)	Serving Size	Cooking Time
baked	until flaky and moist.	carbs, 21g protein, 1g fat, 245mg potassium	(85g)	minutes
Crab, steamed	Steam until meat is opaque and tender.	84 calories, 0g carbs, 17g protein, 1g fat, 250mg potassium	3 oz (85g)	5-7 minutes
Lobster, boiled	Boil until shell turns bright red.	76 calories, 0g carbs, 16g protein, 1g fat, 230mg potassium	3 oz (85g)	7-10 minutes per pound
Shrimp, boiled	Boil until shrimp are opaque and pink.	84 calories, 0g carbs, 20g protein, 1g fat, 190mg potassium	3 oz (85g)	2-3 minutes

Ingredient	Cooking Instructions	Nutritional Information (per serving)	Serving Size	Cooking Time
Clams, steamed	Steam until shells open.	126 calories, 4g carbs, 22g protein, 2g fat, 320mg potassium	3 oz (85g)	5-10 minutes
Scallop, pan-seared	Sear over high heat until golden and opaque.	95 calories, 0g carbs, 20g protein, 1g fat, 205mg potassium	3 oz (85g)	2-3 minutes per side

These meats and protein sources are great options for those managing their potassium intake through diet. When preparing these proteins, keeping seasonings simple and avoiding high-potassium ingredients like tomato sauces or potassium-rich spices will ensure that your meals remain low in potassium. Regular consultations with a dietitian or nutritionist can provide further guidance tailored to your specific health needs.

Dairy and Alternatives

Item	Ingredient	Serving Size	Potassium Content (per serving)	Nutritional Information	Cooking/Preparation Time
1. Rice Milk	Milled rice, water	1 cup	25-50 mg	120 calories, 1g protein	Ready to drink
2. Almond Milk	Almonds, water	1 cup	50 mg	30-50 calories, 1g protein	Ready to drink
3. Coconut Milk	Coconut cream, water	1 cup	50-100 mg	450 calories, 4.6g protein	Ready to drink
4. Soy Milk	Soybeans, water	1 cup	80-100 mg	80-100 calories, 7g protein	Ready to drink
5. Low Fat Cream	Milk, cream	1 ounce	26 mg	30 calories, 2g protein	Ready to use

Item	Ingredient	Serving Size	Potassium Content (per serving)	Nutritional Information	Cooking/Preparation Time
Cheese					
6. Non-Dairy Whipped Topping	Vegetable oils, water	2 tablespoons	0-10 mg	25 calories, 0g protein	Ready to use
7. Nonfat Cottage Cheese	Skim milk, cream, salt	1/2 cup	100 mg	90 calories, 11g protein	Ready to eat
8. Mozzarella (part-skim)	Part-skim milk, enzymes	1 ounce	24 mg	70 calories, 7g protein	Ready to eat
9. Swiss Cheese (low	Part-skim milk,	1 ounce	30 mg	108 calories, 8g protein	Ready to eat

Item	Ingredient	Serving Size	Potassium Content (per serving)	Nutritional Information	Cooking/Preparation Time
sodium)	enzymes				
10. Greek Yogurt (non-fat)	Skim milk, live cultures	100g	50-60 mg	59 calories, 10g protein	Ready to eat
11. Sherbet	Milk, sugar, flavoring	1/2 cup	40-60 mg	140 calories, 1g protein	Ready to eat
12. Lactose-Free Milk	Lactose-free milk	1 cup	90-120 mg	100 calories, 8g protein	Ready to drink
13. Cream (light)	Milk, cream	1 tablespoon	10 mg	29 calories, 0.5g protein	Ready to use

Item	Ingredient	Serving Size	Potassium Content (per serving)	Nutritional Information	Cooking/Preparation Time
14. Tofu (soft)	Soybeans, water, coagulant	1/2 cup	75 mg	94 calories, 10g protein	Ready to eat or cook
15. Non-Dairy Creamer	Vegetable oil, syrup, water	1 tablespoon	10-20 mg	20 calories, 0g protein	Ready to use
16. Hemp Milk	Hemp seeds, water	1 cup	20-40 mg	60-80 calories, 3g protein	Ready to drink
17. Oat Milk	Oats, water	1 cup	80-100 mg	120 calories, 3g protein	Ready to drink
18. Goat Cheese (soft)	Goat milk, culture, enzymes	1 ounce	20-30 mg	75 calories, 5g protein	Ready to eat

Item	Ingredient	Serving Size	Potassium Content (per serving)	Nutritional Information	Cooking/Preparation Time
19. Blue Cheese (crumbled)	Milk, cultures, enzymes	1 ounce	30-40 mg	100 calories, 6g protein	Ready to eat
20. Ricotta (low-fat)	Whey, milk, vinegar	1/4 cup	30-40 mg	40 calories, 3g protein	Ready to eat

This table provides a variety of dairy and non-dairy options suitable for individuals managing their potassium intake. Each item is carefully selected to ensure it is low in potassium, thus helping maintain safe potassium levels while still enjoying a range of tasty and nutritious food choices. The listed preparation times denote whether the item is ready to eat or drink straight from the package, or if minimal preparation is needed.

Snacks and Miscellaneous

For individuals managing their potassium intake, choosing the right snacks can be crucial to maintaining a balanced diet while still enjoying diverse and satisfying options.

Snack	Ingredients	Preparation Instructions	Nutritional Information	Serving Size	Cooking/Preparation Time
Apple Chips	Fresh apples	Slice apples thinly, remove seeds, bake at 200°F until crisp.	95 kcal, Potassium: 100 mg	1 apple	2-3 hours
Rice Cakes	Puffed rice	Available pre-made	35 kcal, Potassium: 29 mg	1 cake	Ready to eat

Snack	Ingredients	Preparation Instructions	Nutritional Information	Serving Size	Cooking/Preparation Time
Popcorn	Popcorn kernels, olive oil	Air pop the kernels, drizzle with a small amount of olive oil.	31 kcal, Potassium: 26 mg	1 cup popped	5 minutes
Cucumber Slices	Cucumber	Slice cucumber thinly.	16 kcal, Potassium: 76 mg	1/2 cucumber	2 minutes
Carrot Sticks	Carrots	Peel carrots, cut into sticks.	25 kcal, Potassium: 80 mg	1 carrot	5 minutes

Snack	Ingredients	Preparation Instructions	Nutritional Information	Serving Size	Cooking/Preparation Time
Breadsticks	Flour, water, yeast, salt	Mix ingredients, knead dough, shape into sticks, and bake.	41 kcal, Potassium: 16 mg	1 stick	18 minutes baking
Boiled Eggs	Eggs	Boil eggs for 10 minutes, cool and peel.	78 kcal, Potassium: 63 mg	1 egg	12 minutes
Unsalted Pretzels	Flour, water, yeast, salt	Mix, shape, boil briefly, and bake until golden.	108 kcal, Potassium: 20 mg	30 grams	25 minutes

Snack	Ingredients	Preparation Instructions	Nutritional Information	Serving Size	Cooking/Preparation Time
Cherry Tomatoes	Cherry tomatoes	Serve fresh.	3 kcal, Potassium: 40 mg	1 tomato	Ready to eat
Homemade Fruit Salad	Apples, pears, berries	Chop fruit and mix.	85 kcal, Potassium: 55 mg per 100 grams	100 grams	10 minutes
Zucchini Chips	Zucchini, olive oil	Slice zucchini, toss with oil, bake until crisp.	50 kcal, Potassium: 150 mg	1 zucchini	45 minutes
Oat Cookies	Oats, banana, apple sauce	Mix ingredients, shape into cookies,	50 kcal, Potassium: 30 mg	1 cookie	15 minutes

Snack	Ingredients	Preparation Instructions	Nutritional Information	Serving Size	Cooking/Preparation Time
		bake.			
Roasted Chickpeas	Chickpeas, olive oil, paprika	Roast chickpeas with oil and spices until crispy.	46 kcal, Potassium: 42 mg	30 grams	30 minutes
Celery Sticks	Celery	Cut celery into sticks.	6 kcal, Potassium: 32 mg	1 stalk	2 minutes
Pita Bread with Hummus	Pita bread, chickpeas, tahini	Blend chickpeas with tahini, serve with pita.	275 kcal, Potassium: 176 mg	1 pita, 2 tbsp hummus	5 minutes prep
Watermelon	Watermelon	Cut watermel	30 kcal, Potassium	1 cup	5 minutes

Snack	Ingredients	Preparation Instructions	Nutritional Information	Serving Size	Cooking/Preparation Time
Cubes		on into cubes.	m: 112 mg		
Unsalted Nuts	Almonds, cashews	Serve raw or toasted.	160 kcal, Potassium: 200 mg	1 oz	Ready to eat
Apple and Cheese	Apple, low-potassium cheese	Slice apple and cheese, serve together.	122 kcal, Potassium: 42 mg	1 apple, 1 oz cheese	5 minutes
Pear Slices with Ricotta	Pear, ricotta cheese	Slice pear, spread ricotta on top.	85 kcal, Potassium: 92 mg	1 pear, 1 tbsp ricotta	5 minutes
Vegetable Soup	Broth, mixed vegetables (low	Simmer vegetables in broth until	70 kcal, Potassium: 55 mg	1 cup	30 minutes

Snack	Ingredients	Preparation Instructions	Nutritional Information	Serving Size	Cooking/Preparation Time
	potassium)	tender.			

These snacks provide a variety of tastes and textures that cater to different preferences and dietary needs, ensuring that maintaining a low-potassium diet doesn't mean sacrificing enjoyment or variety in your snacking habits.

Foods High in Potassium to Avoid

Fruits to Avoid

When managing a low potassium diet, particularly for individuals concerned with lectins (a type of protein that can be difficult to digest and may cause inflammatory responses), certain fruits should be avoided due to their high potassium and lectin content.

Fruit	Potassium Content	Lectin Content	Reason to Avoid
Bananas	High	Moderate	Bananas are very high in potassium and contain lectin, which can exacerbate issues for those with kidney problems and digestive sensitivities.
Avocados	Very High	High	Avocados are extremely high in potassium and also rich in lectins,

Fruit	Potassium Content	Lectin Content	Reason to Avoid
			making them unsuitable for those on low-potassium and low-lectin diets.
Kiwi	High	Moderate	Kiwi fruits, while nutritious, contain a significant amount of potassium and lectins, potentially leading to digestive issues for sensitive individuals.
Melons	High	Moderate	Melons like cantaloupe and honeydew are high in both potassium and lectins, which can interfere with digestive health and potassium balance.
Oranges	High	Moderate	Oranges and other citrus fruits are high in potassium and contain

Fruit	Potassium Content	Lectin Content	Reason to Avoid
			lectins, making them less ideal for those managing their potassium intake and lectin sensitivity.
Mangoes	Moderate	Moderate	Mangoes have a moderate amount of potassium and lectins, which might contribute to digestive discomfort in susceptible individuals.
Grapes	Moderate	Moderate	Grapes are moderately high in potassium and contain lectins, which can pose a risk for those with kidney conditions or those sensitive to lectins.
Papayas	Moderate	Moderate	Papayas contain a moderate level of potassium and lectins, which may cause digestive issues for some people.

Fruit	Potassium Content	Lectin Content	Reason to Avoid
Pomegranates	High	Moderate	Pomegranates are high in potassium and contain lectins, potentially leading to health complications for those requiring strict potassium management.
Dates	Very High	Moderate	Dates are extremely high in potassium and have moderate lectin content, making them unsuitable for a low-potassium, low-lectin diet.
Figs	High	Moderate	Figs, while rich in nutrients, are also high in potassium and lectins, which can exacerbate health issues for individuals on restricted diets.
Prunes	Very High	Moderate	Prunes and prune juice are very high in potassium

Fruit	Potassium Content	Lectin Content	Reason to Avoid
			and contain lectins, posing a risk to those with kidney issues or those who are lectin-sensitive.
Coconuts	High	Moderate	Coconuts and coconut products are high in potassium and contain lectin, potentially aggravating for those managing their intake of these compounds.
Dried Apricots	Very High	Moderate	Dried apricots are particularly high in potassium and have a moderate lectin content, making them a poor choice for those on a low-potassium diet.
Raisins	Very High	Moderate	Raisins, like other dried fruits, concentrate

Fruit	Potassium Content	Lectin Content	Reason to Avoid
			potassium and lectins, which can be detrimental for those needing to control these intakes.
Tomatoes	Moderate	High	Although technically a fruit, tomatoes are moderate in potassium but high in lectins, often advised to be avoided in low-lectin diets.
Bell Peppers	Moderate	High	Like tomatoes, bell peppers are fruits that are moderate in potassium and high in lectins, problematic for sensitive digestive systems.
Passion Fruit	High	Moderate	Passion fruit has a high potassium content and moderate lectins, which can be a concern for those monitoring these

Fruit	Potassium Content	Lectin Content	Reason to Avoid
			dietary components.
Persimmons	High	Moderate	Persimmons are high in potassium and contain lectins, making them unsuitable for those who need to limit these in their diet.
Plums	High	Moderate	Plums and their dried form (prunes) are high in both potassium and lectins, necessitating caution in consumption for those with dietary restrictions.

Avoiding these fruits can help individuals manage conditions that benefit from low potassium and low lectin diets, such as kidney disease, cardiovascular issues, and digestive sensitivities. It's essential for individuals on such diets to consult healthcare providers to ensure nutritional balance and health safety.

Vegetables to Avoid

When managing a diet that is both low in potassium and lectins, it's important to be mindful of certain vegetables that are typically high in these compounds. Lectins are a type of protein that can bind to cell membranes and are thought to have a range of effects on health, from inflammatory responses to digestive issues. Potassium, while crucial for bodily functions, can be harmful in excessive amounts, especially for individuals with kidney issues or those who need to control their potassium levels for other health reasons.

Vegetable	High in Potassium	Contains Lectins	Why to Avoid
Potatoes	Yes	Yes	High in potassium which can exacerbate kidney problems and contain lectins that may affect gut health.
Tomatoes	Yes	Yes	Contain both solanine (a lectin-like substance) and high potassium levels, potentially impacting kidney function and inflammatory processes.

Vegetable	High in Potassium	Contains Lectins	Why to Avoid
Eggplants	Yes	Yes	Similar to tomatoes, eggplants are high in solanine and potassium, which can contribute to inflammation and are problematic for kidney health.
Spinach	Yes	Moderate	Extremely high in potassium and contains some lectins, which can affect digestive health and potassium balance.
Sweet Potatoes	Yes	Yes	Although nutritious, they are high in both potassium and lectin, making them unsuitable for those managing these intakes.
Peppers	Yes	Yes	Contains capsaicin and lectins, which can be irritating to the gut, and high potassium content.

Vegetable	High in Potassium	Contains Lectins	Why to Avoid
Zucchini	Moderate	Yes	Zucchini is moderate in potassium and high in lectins, which can be troublesome for digestive health.
Pumpkin	Moderate	Yes	Contains moderate amounts of potassium and lectins, which can interfere with nutrient absorption and kidney health.
Squash	Moderate	Yes	Winter squashes are moderate in potassium and contain lectins that can contribute to inflammatory issues.
Beets	Yes	Moderate	High in potassium and contain moderate lectin levels, affecting kidney function and blood sugar regulation.

Vegetable	High in Potassium	Contains Lectins	Why to Avoid
Swiss Chard	Yes	Moderate	Very high in potassium and contains lectins, posing risks to those with kidney issues and potentially causing digestive discomfort.
Parsnips	Yes	Moderate	High in potassium and contain lectins, which can impact those with sensitivities or kidney health concerns.
Asparagus	Moderate	Moderate	Contains moderate levels of both potassium and lectins, which may affect kidney function and digestive health.
Kale	Moderate	Yes	High in both potassium and lectins, kale can influence thyroid function and kidney health adversely.
Radishes	Moderate	Yes	Though lower in potassium than some other vegetables,

Vegetable	High in Potassium	Contains Lectins	Why to Avoid
			radishes contain lectins, which can irritate the gut lining.
Artichokes	Yes	Yes	High in potassium and contain lectin proteins, which can complicate health issues related to kidney function and gut health.
Okra	Moderate	Yes	Contains moderate potassium and high lectins, known for causing digestive disturbances.
Collard Greens	Yes	Moderate	High in potassium and contain lectins, making them potentially harmful for kidney health and digestion.
Fennel	Moderate	Moderate	Although lower in lectins, it's moderate in potassium and can contribute to excessive intake if not monitored.

Vegetable	High in Potassium	Contains Lectins	Why to Avoid
Leeks	Moderate	Moderate	Moderate in both potassium and lectins, which could contribute to digestive issues and affect those with kidney disease.

This table should serve as a guideline for those who need to limit both potassium and lectin in their diet, providing a clear indication of which vegetables might best be avoided to maintain health and wellness.

Protein Foods to Avoid

When managing a low potassium diet, particularly for those who also seek to reduce lectins—a type of protein believed by some to cause inflammation and digestive issues—it is important to identify protein foods that are high in potassium and contain significant amounts of lectins.

Protein Food	Reasons to Avoid	High in Potassium	High in Lectins	Additional Notes
Red Kidney Beans	Can cause digestive distress and are very high in potassium.	Yes	Yes	Should be well-cooked to reduce lectin content, but still high in potassium.
Lima Beans	High lectin content can lead to gastrointestinal issues.	Yes	Yes	Also high in potassium, making them doubly unsuitable.
Soybeans	Contain phytoestrogens	Yes	Yes	Often genetically

Protein Food	Reasons to Avoid	High in Potassium	High in Lectins	Additional Notes
	and significant lectins.			modified; high in both potassium and lectins.
Lentils	Although nutritious, they are rich in lectins and potassium.	Yes	Yes	Require thorough cooking to lower lectin levels.
Split Peas	High in lectins, which can interfere with nutrient absorption.	Yes	Yes	Also high in potassium, which can be problematic for kidney health.
Chickpeas	Can cause bloating and gas due to lectins.	Yes	Yes	Also contain a considerable amount of potassium.
Black Beans	High lectin content may	Yes	Yes	Potassium levels are also

Protein Food	Reasons to Avoid	High in Potassium	High in Lectins	Additional Notes
	lead to gastrointestinal discomfort.			a concern.
Navy Beans	Contain lectins that can affect the gut barrier.	Yes	Yes	High in potassium, not recommended for those managing their levels.
Peanuts	Lectins in peanuts can be pro-inflammatory.	Moderate	Yes	Also moderately high in potassium.
Almonds	While nutritious, almonds have moderate lectin and potassium levels.	Moderate	Yes	Better if soaked or sprouted to reduce lectin content.
Walnuts	Contain moderate	Moderate	Yes	Also contain potassium,

Protein Food	Reasons to Avoid	High in Potassium	High in Lectins	Additional Notes
	amounts of lectins.			though less than other nuts.
Sunflower Seeds	Lectins present can contribute to inflammatory responses.	Moderate	Yes	Moderate in potassium, caution is advised.
Quinoa	Contains saponins and lectins which can irritate the gut.	Moderate	Yes	Also has moderate potassium levels.
Tofu	High in both potassium and lectins, can impact thyroid health.	Yes	Moderate	Particularly problematic for those with thyroid issues.
Tempeh	Fermented soy product, still retains some	Yes	Moderate	High in potassium as well.

Protein Food	Reasons to Avoid	High in Potassium	High in Lectins	Additional Notes
	lectins.			
Pumpkin Seeds	Contain lectins, though less than other seeds.	Moderate	Yes	Potassium levels are also considerable.
Chia Seeds	High in lectins, can cause bloating and gas.	Moderate	Yes	Also has moderate potassium content.
Turkey	Higher potassium content than other meats.	Yes	No	Generally low in lectins but high in potassium.
Pork	Higher potassium levels in some cuts.	Yes	No	Low in lectins but not suitable for low potassium diets.
Beef	Some cuts are high in potassium,	Yes	No	Low in lectins but varies in potassium

Protein Food	Reasons to Avoid	High in Potassium	High in Lectins	Additional Notes
	affecting kidney load.			content by cut.

When following a low potassium, low lectin diet, it's crucial to consider both the potassium and lectin content of foods. This table serves as a guide for those who need to manage their dietary intake carefully due to health conditions such as kidney disease, cardiovascular concerns, or digestive sensitivities. By avoiding these foods, individuals can help mitigate health risks associated with high potassium levels and reduce potential digestive discomfort from lectins.

Dairy Products to Avoid

When managing a diet low in potassium, it is crucial to be aware of dairy products that are high in this mineral, as they can quickly contribute to exceeding the recommended daily intake.

Below is a table of 20 dairy products that are typically high in potassium and should be avoided or limited by those following a low-potassium diet. This list is particularly useful for individuals also trying to adhere to a low lectin diet, as some dairy products can be problematic in this regard as well.

Dairy Product	Potassium Content	Reason to Avoid
Milk (Whole)	366 mg per cup	High in potassium and lectins, which can affect digestive health.
Milk (Skim)	382 mg per cup	Similar potassium levels to whole milk; lectins remain even after fat removal.
Yogurt (Plain)	573 mg per cup	Very high in potassium and can contain additives increasing lectin content.

Dairy Product	Potassium Content	Reason to Avoid
Yogurt (Low-fat)	531 mg per cup	Slightly lower in fat but still high in potassium and potentially high in lectins.
Condensed Milk	371 mg per 1/2 cup	Concentrated milk is high in potassium and lectins, potentially exacerbating digestive issues.
Evaporated Milk	419 mg per cup	High in potassium and contains dairy lectins that might contribute to inflammation.
Cream	104 mg per tablespoon	Moderate potassium content but high in fat and lectins.
Sour Cream	73 mg per tablespoon	Although lower in potassium, still contains lectins that can be disruptive to gut health.
Buttermilk	370 mg per cup	High in potassium and contains lectins, which are problematic for those sensitive to dairy.
Cottage Cheese	206 mg per 1/2 cup	Contains a significant amount of potassium and lectins that can affect those with gut sensitivity.

Dairy Product	Potassium Content	Reason to Avoid
Cream Cheese	98 mg per ounce	Lower in potassium but still contains lectins and fats that are problematic for some.
Ricotta Cheese	155 mg per 1/2 cup	Moderate potassium content, but high in lectins that may cause digestive discomfort.
Cheddar Cheese	28 mg per ounce	Low in potassium but high in saturated fats and lectins, which can impact cardiovascular and gut health.
Swiss Cheese	22 mg per ounce	Low in potassium yet contains lectins and fats that may not be ideal for everyone.
Mozzarella Cheese	18 mg per ounce	Very low in potassium but contains lectins, which can contribute to inflammation.
Goat Cheese	39 mg per ounce	Relatively low in potassium but high in lectins, affecting those with lactose intolerance or lectin sensitivity.

Dairy Product	Potassium Content	Reason to Avoid
Parmesan Cheese	24 mg per tablespoon	Low in potassium but high in lectins, potentially irritating for the digestive system.
Feta Cheese	14 mg per ounce	Very low in potassium but still contains lectins that might cause bloating and gas.
Processed Cheese Slices	150-200 mg per slice	Varying levels of potassium and high in processed ingredients and lectins.
Kefir	150 mg per 100 ml	Lower in lactose but still high in potassium and can contain lectins that disrupt gut health.

For individuals following a diet that requires low potassium intake and low lectins, avoiding these dairy products can help manage both potassium levels and reduce the intake of lectins, which are known to cause digestive and inflammatory issues for some people. This careful management can aid in maintaining better overall health and well-being, especially for those with specific dietary sensitivities or chronic health conditions.

Other Foods

When managing a low potassium diet, it's crucial to be mindful of certain foods that are naturally high in potassium. This is particularly important for individuals with conditions that require potassium regulation such as kidney disease or those on certain medications. Beyond the typical fruits and vegetables commonly known for their high potassium content, other food groups including nuts, seeds, and chocolates also contribute significant amounts of potassium and should be consumed cautiously or avoided.

Food Item	Reason to Avoid	Average Potassium Content	Common Serving Size
Almonds	High in potassium, may contribute to hyperkalemia in susceptible individuals.	705 mg	1 oz (about 23 nuts)
Walnuts	Similarly high in potassium, potentially dangerous for those with kidney issues.	441 mg	1 oz (about 14 halves)

Food Item	Reason to Avoid	Average Potassium Content	Common Serving Size
Hazelnuts	High potassium content can exacerbate health conditions requiring potassium management.	634 mg	1 oz (about 21 nuts)
Cashews	Potassium levels are considerable, posing a risk for those on restricted diets.	660 mg	1 oz (about 18 nuts)
Pistachios	Contain significant potassium, making them unsuitable for low potassium diets.	295 mg	1 oz (about 49 nuts)
Brazil Nuts	Extremely high in potassium, to be avoided by those monitoring their intake.	659 mg	1 oz (about 6 nuts)
Pumpkin Seeds	High potassium content could lead to complications in potassium-sensitive	588 mg	1 oz

Food Item	Reason to Avoid	Average Potassium Content	Common Serving Size
	conditions.		
Sunflower Seeds	While nutritious, they are high in potassium and may not be suitable for everyone.	850 mg	1 oz
Flaxseeds	Contain high levels of potassium, which might not align with dietary restrictions.	813 mg	1 oz
Chia Seeds	Despite their health benefits, their high potassium content can be a concern.	407 mg	1 oz
Milk Chocolate	Contains moderate levels of potassium, better avoided on strict low potassium diets.	203 mg	1 oz
Dark Chocolate	Higher potassium content than milk	372 mg	1 oz

Food Item	Reason to Avoid	Average Potassium Content	Common Serving Size
	chocolate, risky for those managing intake.		
Baking Chocolate	Used in many desserts, it has a high potassium content and should be used sparingly.	830 mg	1 oz
Cocoa Powder	Very high in potassium, a concern for anyone on a potassium-restricted diet.	1317 mg	1 oz
Pecans	High in potassium, not ideal for low potassium diet adherence.	410 mg	1 oz (about 19 halves)
Macadamia Nuts	Rich in potassium, problematic for those needing to control their levels.	368 mg	1 oz (about 10-12 nuts)
Pine Nuts	Elevated potassium levels make these nuts unsuitable for some diets.	597 mg	1 oz

Food Item	Reason to Avoid	Average Potassium Content	Common Serving Size
Hemp Seeds	They contain a significant amount of potassium, which can affect some health conditions.	370 mg	1 oz
Sesame Seeds	High in potassium, should be limited or avoided in low potassium diets.	468 mg	1 oz
Coconut	While popular, coconut is high in potassium and should be consumed in moderation.	356 mg	1 oz shredded

This table not only highlights the potassium content in these foods but also emphasizes the necessity for individuals on potassium-restricted diets to avoid or limit their intake to maintain healthy potassium levels. By focusing on this aspect of diet management, individuals can better prevent the complications associated with high potassium levels, such as hyperkalemia.

Tips for Eating Out

Choosing Low Potassium Options at Restaurants

Eating out while managing a low potassium diet can be challenging, but with the right knowledge and strategies, it is entirely possible to enjoy a meal at a restaurant without compromising on dietary restrictions. The key is preparation and knowing which menu items are typically low in potassium.

When dining out, it's beneficial to select restaurants that offer a variety of meal options and are willing to customize dishes upon request. Fast food restaurants might be less accommodating compared to sit-down restaurants where chefs can often prepare meals to order without certain ingredients.

One effective strategy is to review the restaurant's menu online before visiting. Many restaurants now provide nutritional information on their websites, which can help identify dishes with lower potassium content. If the information isn't available online, consider calling the restaurant ahead of time to discuss your dietary needs.

This can prevent any surprises and ensure the staff is prepared to accommodate your requests.

When ordering, it's wise to focus on grilled or roasted meats and fish, as these are generally prepared without added sauces or seasonings that might contain high levels of potassium. It's also important to ask for no added salt, as salt substitutes are often high in potassium. Instead of starchy sides like potatoes or dishes that include tomato sauces, opt for steamed vegetables like green beans, cauliflower, or peppers, and always ask for sauces and dressings to be served on the side so you can control the amount you consume.

Bread can be a good option, but it's best to avoid whole grain and wheat varieties as they are higher in potassium. Choose white bread or rolls instead. For salads, stick with leafy greens like lettuce or spinach, and add items like cucumbers, radishes, and onions, avoiding higher potassium vegetables like tomatoes, avocados, and nuts.

Beverage choices should also be considered carefully. It's best to avoid or limit the intake of beverages like milk or orange juice, which are high in potassium. Opt for water, lemonade, or other fruit juices that are lower in potassium, such as apple or cranberry.

For dessert, avoid fruits like bananas, oranges, or kiwi. Instead, look for alternatives like apple pie, lemon sorbet, or cakes made without chocolate or nuts.

Lastly, don't hesitate to ask the server to relay your dietary needs to the kitchen and double-check how the food is prepared. Restaurants are accustomed to handling a variety of dietary requests and can often provide the necessary accommodations to ensure you have a safe and enjoyable dining experience. By staying informed and making careful choices, dining out can still be a pleasurable part of your lifestyle while managing a low potassium diet.

Fast Food and Low Potassium Choices

Navigating fast food menus while adhering to a low potassium diet requires a strategic approach, as fast food is typically rich in potassium due to ingredients like tomatoes, potatoes, and processed meats. However, with careful selection and modifications, it is possible to enjoy eating out without significantly disrupting potassium levels.

One effective strategy is to focus on simple grilled or broiled items, such as grilled chicken sandwiches or plain burgers without additives like cheese or sauces, which often contain higher potassium. Requesting the removal of high-potassium toppings such as tomato slices and avoiding condiments like ketchup, which is high in potassium, can also help manage intake.

Salads from fast food chains can be a good option, but it's important to be selective with ingredients. Opting for salads without nuts, seeds, or cheese and asking for a low-potassium dressing or simply using lemon juice or vinegar can maintain low potassium levels. Additionally, avoiding high-potassium vegetables like avocados and opting for greens, cucumbers, and shredded carrots can make salads safer.

For side dishes, skipping French fries and opting for a side salad or apple slices can dramatically reduce potassium intake. If salads are not an option, requesting customizations like a baked potato without the skin can also be a viable alternative, as most of the potassium in potatoes is found in the skin.

When it comes to beverages, it's best to stick with water, plain coffee, or iced tea instead of fruit juices or milkshakes, which are generally high in potassium. Soda is typically low in potassium but should be consumed in moderation due to other health considerations like high sugar content.

Breads and cereals are generally safe in moderation. When selecting sandwiches, choosing options with white or refined bread instead of whole grains can help manage potassium levels as whole grains are typically higher in potassium.

In terms of desserts, opting for items like cookies or ice cream in small quantities can be suitable as these are typically lower in potassium than desserts containing nuts, chocolate, or large amounts of dairy.

It's also advisable to consult nutritional information that many fast food chains provide online or in-store. Many chains offer detailed nutritional guides that list potassium content, allowing for more informed decisions.

Ultimately, maintaining a low potassium diet while eating fast food is about making informed choices and understanding the composition of different foods. By focusing on simple, minimally processed foods and avoiding high-potassium additives, individuals can enjoy the convenience of fast food without compromising their health needs.

Monitoring and Managing Potassium Intake

How to Track Your Potassium Intake

Tracking potassium intake is critical for individuals who need to manage their potassium levels due to health conditions like chronic kidney disease, heart problems, or those taking certain medications that affect potassium balance. Effective monitoring involves several strategies that ensure dietary potassium does not exceed recommended limits, and each plays a vital role in maintaining health and preventing complications.

One of the first steps in tracking potassium intake is understanding the potassium content in foods. Resources such as the "Low Potassium Food List" provide detailed information on the potassium levels in various foods, helping individuals make informed choices about what to include in their diet. Using such lists as a reference, one can plan meals and snacks carefully, ensuring that high-potassium foods are minimized or avoided.

For accurate tracking, maintaining a food diary is highly beneficial. In this diary, every consumed item is recorded along with its portion size and potassium content, which can typically be found using nutrition labels or reliable online nutritional databases. By reviewing this diary regularly, individuals can assess their daily and weekly potassium intake and make necessary adjustments to stay within their dietary limits.

In addition to manual tracking, there are numerous digital tools and apps available that can simplify this process. These applications often feature extensive food databases that provide instant information on the potassium content of most foods, including restaurant dishes and pre-packaged foods. Some apps also allow users to set daily potassium intake goals and track their progress toward these goals, alerting them when they are approaching or exceeding their recommended potassium limit.

Another aspect of monitoring potassium intake is understanding how food preparation techniques can affect potassium levels. For example, leaching vegetables by cutting them into small pieces and soaking them in water before cooking can help reduce their potassium content. Being aware of such techniques and applying them in meal preparation can further aid in managing intake.

Regular consultations with a healthcare provider are essential for those managing potassium intake for health reasons. These consultations can provide opportunities to discuss the effectiveness of current dietary strategies and make adjustments based on blood test results. Healthcare providers can also offer additional guidance and support, such as referring patients to a dietitian who specializes in managing diets for specific health conditions.

Lastly, educating oneself continuously about potassium management through books, reputable websites, and support groups can provide additional tips and strategies. Engaging with others who are also managing their potassium intake can offer practical advice and moral support, making the process more manageable.

By combining these strategies—using detailed food lists, keeping a food diary, utilizing digital tools, applying food preparation techniques, consulting with healthcare professionals, and engaging in ongoing education—individuals can effectively track and manage their potassium intake. This comprehensive approach not only helps in adhering to a low-potassium diet but also supports overall health and well-being.

Adjusting Potassium Intake Based on Medical Needs

Adjusting potassium intake based on medical needs is a critical aspect of managing various health conditions, particularly those related to kidney function and cardiovascular health. Proper potassium management can help prevent both high and low potassium levels, each of which carries its own set of risks and complications.

For individuals with chronic kidney disease (CKD) or those on dialysis, the kidneys may not be able to filter potassium effectively, which can lead to hyperkalemia. Hyperkalemia increases the risk of developing dangerous heart arrhythmias and other cardiac problems. Conversely, certain medications and other health conditions may cause hypokalemia, or low levels of potassium, which can lead to muscle weakness, cramps, and cardiac disturbances.

The specific amount of potassium appropriate for an individual can vary widely based on their overall health, kidney function, and the medications they are taking. Therefore, it's essential for patients to work closely with healthcare providers to determine their ideal daily potassium intake. This process often involves regular blood tests to monitor potassium levels and adjust dietary intake as needed.

For those advised to follow a low potassium diet, understanding which foods are high in potassium and which are low is vital. High-potassium foods like bananas, oranges, potatoes, and tomatoes should be limited or avoided. Instead, individuals can focus on low-potassium choices such as apples, berries, carrots, and green beans. Comprehensive resources such as the "Low Potassium Food List" are invaluable for making informed choices about dietary intake.

Meal planning is also an integral part of managing dietary potassium. By planning meals in advance, individuals can ensure a balanced intake of nutrients while keeping their potassium levels within a safe range. This might include using specialized nutrition tracking apps or tools that help in logging and analyzing food intake.

Adjustments in diet may also need to be responsive to changes in medication or the progression of underlying health conditions. For instance, if a patient's kidney function declines, they may need to further restrict potassium. Similarly, if they are prescribed a new medication that affects potassium levels, dietary adjustments might be necessary to compensate.

Educational resources and support from dietitians can help patients understand and implement dietary changes effectively. Regular consultations and ongoing education about the role of potassium in the body and how it is impacted by various foods are crucial.

In addition to dietary management, some patients might require medical treatment to manage potassium levels directly. This can include medications that increase potassium excretion or protect the heart from the effects of high potassium.

Ultimately, the goal of adjusting potassium intake based on medical needs is to maintain potassium at a level that supports overall health without leading to additional complications. This requires a coordinated approach involving careful dietary management, regular medical monitoring, and, in some cases, the use of specific medications designed to help control potassium levels.

Conclusion

In conclusion, adopting a low potassium diet with the guidance of resources like the "Low Potassium Food List" can be a transformative step towards better health and well-being for individuals managing conditions such as kidney disease, heart issues, or other potassium-sensitive ailments. By understanding the importance of potassium management and making informed choices about dietary intake, individuals can effectively mitigate the risks associated with abnormal potassium levels.

The comprehensive information provided in resources like the "Low Potassium Food List" empowers individuals to navigate their dietary choices with confidence, offering clear guidelines on which foods to include and which to avoid. From fruits and vegetables to grains, proteins, and snacks, the guide provides a wealth of options tailored to fit within a low potassium diet while still ensuring a diverse and satisfying culinary experience.

Moreover, the benefits of adopting a low potassium diet extend beyond merely managing potassium levels. By focusing on whole, nutrient-rich foods and avoiding processed and high-potassium items, individuals can improve overall nutrition and support better cardiovascular and kidney health. Additionally, the emphasis on mindful eating and meal planning encourages healthier lifestyle habits that can have long-lasting benefits beyond potassium management alone.

However, it's important to recognize that managing potassium intake is not a one-size-fits-all approach. Each individual's dietary needs may vary based on factors such as their underlying health conditions, medications, and personal preferences. Therefore, ongoing communication with healthcare providers, regular monitoring of potassium levels, and flexibility in dietary adjustments are essential components of success.

In the journey towards better health through dietary management, the "Low Potassium Food List" serves as a valuable tool and companion, offering support, guidance, and practical solutions to help individuals achieve their health goals. By embracing the principles of a low potassium diet and making conscientious choices about food intake, individuals can take control of their health and experience improved quality of life.